Get Started w

A Beginners Guide to th
Fat Die

@2014 Small Guides

Table of Contents

Book Description

Finding a diet plan that works for you can be really difficult. There are so many that are out there and all of them claim that they are better than the others and will provide you with the best results. With all of the options that are out there, how do you choose the one that works for you?

If you have tried out many different weight loss and diet plans, you may be tired of working hard and not seeing the results that you need. For those that feel like they are in a rut, the Low Carb High Fat diet may be the answer that you need. Instead of getting on another diet plan that is too difficult to maintain or that sounds like all of the others, the LCHF diet plan will give you some easy steps that you can follow that will help you to lose the weight while still feeling full and satisfied. The best part is that if you are able to follow some of the basic requirements of this diet plan, then you will not have to waste your time with weighing food or counting calories in order to lose the weight.

This guidebook is meant to provide you with the information that you need in order to get started and be successful on the LCHF diet. It provides chapters with information on topics such as:

- What is the Low Carb High Fat Diet
- Beginners difficulties on the LCHF diet
- Foods to eat and foods to avoid on the LCHF diet
- The differences between the LCHF diet and the Atkins Diet
- And some basic tips for getting started.

Check out this guidebook today to learn how easy it can be to lose weight without having to do all of that extra work that is required from other diet plans.

Introduction

If you are tired of all of the endless claims that come from the many diet plans that are out there promising great weight loss even though you haven't lost a thing, then a low carb high fat diet might be just the thing that you are looking for. Instead of forcing you to endlessly watch what you are eating, weigh and measure your food, and count the calories all day long, this diet plan just asks you to limit your carb intake while increasing your consumption of healthy fats. That is it! If you can follow those two simple rules than you are able to avoid all of the hassle that comes with other diet plans, eat until you feel satisfied and still lose weight. This guidebook is meant to provide you with the information that you need to learn more about the LCHF diet and make the decision to include it into your life.

Chapter 1 starts out by giving an overview of what the LCHF diet is. It explains the advantages of this diet plan, how it can help you to lose weight, and how the process of ketosis occurs during an LCHF diet to help you lose weight.

Chapter 2 continues on by explaining some of the difficulties that you may face as a beginner on this diet plan and tells you some things that you can do to avoid those issues.

Chapter 3 goes on to explain what kinds of fats that you should enjoy while on this diet plan in order to lose weight. There is also a section about some of the foods that you should avoid completely on the LCHF diet and which foods you should only have on an occasion.

Chapter 4 talks about how the LCHF diet is different from the Atkins diet while

Chapter 5 This chapter is providing you with a menu for the first 14 days on the LCHF diet to help you to get started.

Take a look through this guidebook to find out all of the information that you need to see great success while on the LCHF diet plan.

Chapter 1—What is LCHF?

With all of the choices that are out there for you to choose from for diet plans, it can be difficult to distinguish one from the other and determine which one will work out the best for your needs. Some diet plans seem really difficult and require you to monitor and record so many different things that it is more work than it is worth. On the other side of things, some diets promise you amazing weight loss results with just taking a pill and not changing up anything else in your daily life; although most of these are just fad diets that cause more harm than good anyway. Somewhere in the middle of these two spectrums is the perfect diet to meet your needs.

If you are looking to get started on a great diet plan you might be interested in the low carb high fat, or LCHF, diet plan. With this diet plan, you will eat fewer carbohydrates in your daily diet and more fats. In addition to this, you will have to limit the amount of starches and sugar that you are consuming as well. Outside of these requirements, you will be able to eat many other great tasting foods without having to count the calories all of the time—just eat until you feel satisfied and you will be able to lose weight. The best part about this diet is that it is not just a fad diet that will not help you out at all or will make you lose weight unsafely. There have been several high quality studies that have been done recently that show how being on a LCHF diet can make it easier for you to control the levels of your blood sugar while still losing weight. This chapter will discuss some of the benefits that you can get from following this diet plan so you can determine if it is the right one for you!

To get started on this diet plan we will start with the basics. You will need to first realize the foods that you are allowed to eat while on this diet plan and the ones that you are supposed to avoid. While following the LCHF diet you are allowed to eat healthy foods such as vegetables, eggs, fish, and meats and some fruits. You are even allowed to eat some natural fats and ones that are found above the ground, such as butter.

The foods that you are supposed to avoid while on this kind of diet plan include anything that would have a lot of carbs in it, sugars, and other starchy foods such as potatoes, rice, pasta, and bread.

While it is impossible to completely cut out all of the carbs that are in your daily diet, it is important that you work to limit them as much as possible on this diet plan and try to eat some other foods that are better for you. In addition, when you are following this kind of diet plan you are allowed to eat whenever you want as long as you are hungry and you can keep eating until you feel full. Do not overeat or eat when you are not hungry, even if it is the traditional time for eating a meal. That is all you have to keep in mind for this diet plan. There is no counting of calories or spending a lot of time weighing out your food to make sure that you are eating the right amount of weight loss.

All the work that you will do for this diet is make sure to keep your carb count low, eat plenty of fats, and just eat when you are hungry and stop when you get full. Also, make sure that you are eating real food that is not processed and does not contain a ton of sugar and other bad things that can harm your body and make you gain weight. If you are able to follow these simple rules, then you will find a lot of success with this diet plan.

There are many reasons why this diet plan will work well for keeping you healthy and the weight off and they can also be proven by science. To start with, the LCHF diet plan helps you to avoid starches and sugars in your diet. When you are able to do this, you can stabilize your blood sugar which will keep the levels of your insulin down inside the body. Since insulin is the hormone that stores fat in your body, you will be able to effectively increase the amount of fat that your body is burning while still feeling like you are full after eating a meal.

There are many different types of foods that you are able to eat while following the LCHF diet. Some of these include foods such as:

- Meat—you can eat any kind of meat that you like including chicken, game meat, pork, and beef. You can even keep the fat on your beef and the skin on the chicken if you would like. It is recommended that you stick with grass fed or organic meat if you are able to for the best results.
- Fish—as with meat, you are able to enjoy any kind of fish that you would like while following this diet plan. Even the fish that are considered fatty, such as herring, mackerel, and salmon can be enjoyed. One thing that you should keep in mind while you are eating fish is that they should not have any breading on them.
- Eggs—eggs are also encouraged while you are following this diet plan and you can prepare them in any method that you prefer. If you are able to, pick out organic eggs for your use.
- High fat, natural fat sauces—cream and butter can be used to help with the cooking process if you would like. While this is different from many other diet plans, it is a great way to make your food taste great and leave you feeling more satiated. Hollandaise and Bearnaise sauces are great options as are olive oil and coconut oil.
- Above ground vegetables—there is a long list of vegetables that are highly encouraged while you are following this diet plan. Some options that you may want to try out include tomatoes, peppers, onions, avocado, lettuce, cucumber, olives, cabbage, zucchini, and broccoli.
- Dairy products—something that is different about this diet plan compared to some of the others is that you should pick the full-fat options of dairy products rather than the low or no fat options. The lower fat milk and dairy product options will often have a lot of sugar, which is not allowed on this diet plan. You should also

be careful of any dairy product that has extra sugar or which has been flavored.

- Nuts—nuts can be consumed on this diet plan as long as you make sure to do so in moderation. Choose a few nuts for a healthy snack rather than your usual candy
- Berries—some berries can be enjoyed as long as you only have them in moderation and if you are not really sensitive to the sugars found in them.

What is the Advantage of LCHF

Now that you know a little bit about the LCHF diet, you may be wondering what some of the advantages of choosing this diet over some of the other diet plans may be. This section is going to discuss some of the great benefits that come with following this diet plan.

1. Losing weight—the first reason that you have chosen this diet plan is that you are probably trying to lose weight. Luckily the LCHF diet can help you out with this. There have been several scientific studies done that show that it is possible to lose weight while following the LCHF diet. The amount that you will be able to lose on this diet plan will vary depending on your circumstances, how much weight you need to lose in the first place, and how well you are able to follow and maintain this diet plan.
2. Blood sugar improvements—in addition to studies being done that prove that you can lose weight on this diet plan, there have been ones done to show that when you follow a low carb diet, you are able to reduce the fasting glucose levels in the body. This is beneficial to the body in keeping your blood sugar levels down, especially if you have prediabetes or diabetes.
3. Blood pressure improvements—many people are suffering from high blood pressure and it is one of the leading risk factors for worse problems such as heart

disease and stroke. It is critical that you find ways to lower your blood pressure in order to avoid these serious cardiovascular diseases. The LCHF diet is effective in lowering the blood pressure of those who are overweight or obese.

4. Insulin resistance reduction—those who are suffering from metabolic syndrome know how it is to deal with insulin resistance on a regular basis. Not only can this cause some issues with your blood pressure, there is also a correlation between cardiovascular disease and insulin resistance. Luckily, there have been studies done that show that by restricting the amounts of carbs that you are consuming, such as what is done in the LCHF diet, you will be able to significantly lower your insulin resistance, especially when compared to a diet that requires you to limit your fat intake instead.

5. Lower insulin levels—lowering your insulin levels can be important to those who are dealing with prediabetes, insulin resistance, and diabetes. These people would benefit from following a diet that limits the amount of carbs that they consume, such as the LCHF diet, in order to decrease their insulin levels and live healthier lives.

LCHF and Weight Loss

Weight loss is the number one reason why most people decide to go on a weight loss and diet plan. They might be tired of the way that they look and feel and are finally ready to do something to make it better. Or they may be suffering from one of a host of other diseases, such as heart problems, diabetes, high blood pressure, high cholesterol levels, and much more and would greatly benefit from losing some weight to get these health issues in check. No matter the reason that you are trying to lose weight, the LCHF diet is effective in helping you out.

There have been several recent studies conducted that prove that following a diet like the LCHF diet can be beneficial and efficient in helping you to lose weight. To start with, when you limit the amounts of carbs that you are consuming each day, you are helping to keep your insulin levels in check. When insulin is in check, it will be able to release the fat stores that are in your body, making it easier for you to get it out of the body. You will be able to eat foods that contain good and natural fats and lose weight while still feeling satiated.

The best part about this weight loss plan is that you do not have to spend all of your time weighing food or counting calories. Instead, you can just eat whenever you are hungry and stop when you feel full, making sure that the foods that you are eating are healthy and not full of sugars, carbs, and other processed foods. If you can follow these simple steps, you will be able to see some amazing weight loss results.

LCHF and Ketosis

While you are on the LCHF diet, you will be teaching your body how to adapt on ketones all of the time. This can sometimes be difficult for people to get used to in the beginning and you may feel that you are doing something wrong. Feeling extra tired and even a little bit woozy is perfectly normal. After a couple of weeks, things though get back to normal and you will even start to feel a little bit better. Many people who have been able to get through the first little difficulties with running completely on ketones, then you will be able to feel sharper and have an easier time focusing on what is going on.

During ketosis, you might also notice that your exercise program will be a little bit different. For the first couple of days, you may not notice any differences at all and everything will seem normal. After those initial first days, up to a little over a week, you may notice that your performance in the gym will start to decrease and your muscles begin to tire out more quickly. It is important to keep working out whenever you are able to and work as hard as possible to get through the soreness and tiredness. Once you get into the third or fourth week, then your strength is going to start coming back. In fact, you may notice that your workout sessions are getting better and that you will be able to work out longer and lift more weight than ever before.

There are many other effects that you may notice early on when you go into ketosis while on the LCHF diet. To start with, you may notice that you are feeling thirsty all of the time. Your body is trying to get rid of all the bad toxins that are stuck in your body, which is going to take a ton of water to do. Some of those who are going through ketosis will state that they will feel thirsty even if they drink plenty of water. After some time you will get used to this and your body will start to balance out a little bit and the thirst issue will not be as bad.

There are also some breath issues that come into play when you are going through the first couple of weeks during ketosis. Those that are in the process of going through this process may notice that their breath is reminiscent of fruit or even nail polish removers. This is just a little annoyance that you will be able to get through and after just a few weeks you will have this bad breath go away.

You may also notice that your sense of taste, especially in terms of things that are sweet, is that they will be more noticeable. If you were someone who really enjoyed eating a lot of sweets and having sodas before going on the LCHF diet, then you may have become a little too used to the sweetness that is in them. While on the LCHF diet, you are going to have to limit the amounts of sweets and processed foods that you are eating so your taste buds will become unused to them. After being on the LCHF diet for some time, when you eat a sweet, you may notice that things seem so much stronger and sweeter when you go back to them.

These are just a few of the things that you may notice when you go through the ketosis phase on the LCHF diet. It is important to realize that any of the difficulties and troublesome parts that come with this diet will only last for a few weeks. If you can get through the few weeks, you will feel a lot stronger and more alert and will really be able to enjoy the results that come with being on this great diet.

Chapter 2—LCHF and Beginner Difficulties

As with any diet plan, there are going to be some difficulties that you are going to have to get through when you first start out on the LCHF diet. This chapter will discuss the top 8 side effects that can come with this diet plan.

1. Confusion—the first thing that you may notice when you start on the LCHF diet is that you are feeling more confused than normal. This period will usually occur about 3 days into the new diet plan. There are times that you may find that you are feeling half-drunk, staring at walls, or feeling like you are unproductive. This is known as a fogging of the brain and will usually occur because your body and brain are working to learn how to adapt to a life with limited sugar. Since your brain is used to using sugar as its primary form of energy, it can get a little confused and not know what to do when you take that sugar away. This will only last a few days until your body learns how to switch from using the sugar as energy to using fat instead. Just work on getting through this cloud of fog for a few days and you will start to feel really great while on this diet plan.

2. Flu and Fatigue—when you start on a low carb diet, your body might feel like it has gone through a horrible ordeal. Some people will even state that they will feel flu-like symptoms. Some of the symptoms that you may expect include general weakness, muscle cramps, nausea, and headaches all of which can make you not feel well for a few days. This is caused by the fact that your body has become very dependent on using carbs for energy and when you take the carbs away, your body is not sure what to do. The nice thing is that you can plan ahead for this. Instead of starting the diet at the beginning of the week, start on a Thursday so that you can have the weekend to get through these symptoms and start feeling good again.

3. Irritability—some people have found that they get really irritable when they start a low carb diet. This is because your body is trying to get used to not having the foods that it is used to and it can leave you feeling annoyed and irritable at some of the things that are going on. Make sure that when you first start this new diet plan you eat a lot of quality proteins and fresh vegetables. These will provide you with the potassium, manganese, and iron that are critical to helping your mind stay clear and your energy levels to stay high.
4. Strange tastes and smells—ketones are products that are in your body which are byproducts of fat being used as fuel when the carbs are reduced from your diet. This process, known as ketosis, can often result in some smells and tastes that are strange coming from your body. Some people that get on this kind of diet plan will say that they have gotten a tangy or fruity taste inside their mouth along with breath that is strange smelling. Not everyone will have this issue, though it has been shown that those who have type 1 diabetes will be more likely to experience it. Increasing your intake of water and slowly restricting the carbs from your diet can help.
5. Decrease in strength and muscle aches—your body is used to having lots of carbs in order to get the fuel that it needs and keep your energy up. When you take away those carbs, your body will have to switch gears and learn how to deal with using fat for energy instead. This is going to be tough on your body for the first few weeks so you may feel achy and tired until your body adapts. To help limit the amount of aches and pains that you are feeling, you can start out slowly on restricting the carbs instead of getting rid of them completely. Also, for the first few weeks, you may want to be careful about the amounts of intense exercises that you are doing.
6. Constipation—Since the LCHF diet has you cut out many sources of fiber, nuts, legumes, beans, and whole grains, you may start to suffer from constipation.

Luckily, you will still be able to avoid constipation by getting the fiber that you need when you consume a ton of vegetables. This is absolutely required if you want to avoid constipation and to keep your bowel movements normal. Make sure to get as many vegetables into your diet as possible to help avoid this problem.

7. Dehydration—many of the LCHF diets that you can choose from will be known for the diuretic effect that they cause on those that follow them. Dehydration can often happen on these diets since you are losing a lot of nutrients and water while on this diet plan. Make sure that while you are on this diet plan, you drink plenty of water. You will need to drink a minimum of 8 glasses of water or other liquids each day in order to keep your body hydrated and to replace any of the electrolytes that you may be losing through excess peeing and the exercise you do.

8. Depression—your body is going to crave carbs in order to properly function and when you limit the amount of carbs that are in your diet, you may notice an impact in the levels of serotonin in your brain. This means that you may be at risk for a mood imbalance and depression. There are a couple of other foods that you will be able to take in order to keep your serotonin levels up and help you to feel great. One of the best options is turkey, almonds, tuna, salmon, and leafy greens.

Chapter 3—LCHF—Fat and Cholesterol

While you are following the LCHF diet plan, you will be required to limit the amounts of carbs that you are consuming and will instead need to focus on eating fats in your diet instead. This is a lot different from other diet plans that are out there since most of them want you to limit the amounts and types of fats that you are consuming to the point of hardly eating any at all. Getting out of this mindset can be really difficult for some people but it is critical if you want to see the great results that come from an LCHF diet.

The important thing to remember here is that it all matters what kinds of fats you are consuming. Just because you are allowed to eat fats on this diet plan does not mean that you should go out and eat fast food every day and expect to see results. Instead of eating these fats that are bad for you and will just keep the weight on, you will need to make sure to choose fats that are healthy and can keep you feeling your very best.

When you load up on the saturated fats, you are doing nothing good for your body and you are going to end up regretting it in the long run. These bad fats will raise up your cholesterol levels, lead you to becoming obese, can lead to diabetes, and ultimately will lead to heart disease. Take the time to learn about the different kinds of fats so that you can choose the ones that will fill you up and help you to lose the weight that you want while on this diet plan.

What is "forbidden" to eat on LCHF

One thing that you are really going to have to watch out for when you are on any diet plan is which foods to avoid. You are not going to be very successful on the LCHF diet plan if you spend all of your time eating foods that are filled with carbs or other foods that are not allowed on this diet plan. Here are some of the foods that you should make sure that you are avoiding if you want to see success on this diet plan. They include:

- Sugar—the number one thing that you are going to have to stay away from while following an LCHF diet is sugar. This can include anything from breakfast cereals, ice cream, pastries, buns, cakes, chocolate, sports drinks, juice, candy, and sodas. It is also best if you are able to avoid any kind of sweeteners in your food as well.
- Starches—starches must also be avoided if you want to see success on a LCHF diet. Starches can include things like muesli, porridge, potato chips, French fries, potatoes, rice, pasta, and bread. If you decide to have some starches in your diet, you should be sure to pick the whole grain versions if possible, although these should be avoided as well. A little amount of root vegetables can be allowed as well.
- Margarine—there really are no benefits to consuming margarine other than the fact that it helps food to taste a little better. You will be able to get the same taste results from much healthier options. Margarine was developed in order to imitate butter but it has a lot more fat, has been linked to inflammatory diseases, allergies, and asthma, tastes bad, and has no other health benefits.
- Beer—even though it might be fun to go out with friends on an occasion and have a few beers to drink, this should be avoided as much as possible. Beer is full of carbs that can ruin all of your hard work on the LCHF diet. Choose another kind of alcohol if you decide to go out and drink.
- Fruit—while most diets will tell you how important it is to eat a lot of healthy fruits in order to lose weight, it is best to avoid fruits as much as possible while following an LCHF diet plan. This is because fruits are very sweet from their high sugar content. It is fine to eat fruit once in a while, especially with all of the great vitamins

and nutrients that you can get from them, but it is best to treat it as another form of natural candy.

In addition to having some foods that you are not allowed to consume at all while following an LCHF diet plan, there are some foods that you are allowed to eat on an occasion, but you should try to limit them as much as possible. These foods and beverages include:

- Alcohol—it is best to avoid drinking alcohol as much as possible because many of the choices that you can make will contain a lot of extra sugar that is not good for you and will mess up your carb counts. In addition, there are a lot of extra calories in many alcoholic beverages which will make it even more difficult to lose the weight that you want. That being said, some options, such as cocktails, vodka, brandy, whisky, and dry wine, are much better options than beer and should be chosen instead when going out for a drink.
- Dark chocolate—it is fine to consume a little bit of dark chocolate when you are on an LCHF diet, as long as you do so in moderation. When choosing your dark chocolate, make sure that it contains more than 70% cocoa in it.

These are just some of the general guidelines that are necessary to follow while on the LCHF diet. You should try as hard as you can to maintain these requirements in order to get the best results possible. It is important to keep in mind that it is possible to slip up and make mistakes or eat something that is not allowed on this diet plan. Many people who try to stick too hard to a diet plan and do not allow themselves any room for error will find that the diet plan is too difficult. After a while, no matter how hard they try, they will slip up, binge eat, and may not get back on the diet plan at all.

This is why it may be a good idea to set up a "cheat day" during your diet. Once a week you allow yourself to eat a thing or two that are not usually allowed on the diet plan as long as you followed all of the rules and were good during the rest of the week. For example, you may allow yourself to have a small candy bar or a small pop one day if you have been good the rest of the week.

Doing this is great because it lets you work hard all week and reward yourself instead of leaving you deprived all of the time. Just make sure that when you have your cheat day you are not overdoing it. A cheat day is a time for you to enjoy a little something as a reward, not an excuse to eat anything you want and as much of it as you want.

Chapter 4—What is the difference between LCHF and the Atkins Diet

After reading through some of the information that has been presented in this guidebook, you may be wondering what makes this diet plan different from some of the other ones that ask you to limit the amount of carbs that you are consuming in your daily diet. In fact, they may sound very similar and you may be tempted to try out one of the other diet plans that are available. This chapter is going to focus on the differences between a GI diet, LCHF diet, and the Atkins diet.

If you choose to go on a low GI diet, you will have to realize that you are not really limiting the amount of carbs that you are consuming in your daily diet. This is already going against one of the main ideas that is brought up in an LCHF diet plan. Instead of limiting the amount of carbs that you consume, you are instead limiting the type of carbs consumed on a low GI diet. This kind of diet plan asks you to choose carbs that are slow releasing rather than regular carbs in order to slow down the rise in your blood sugars that will occur.

Now comes the Atkins diet. Many people will claim that the Atkins diet and the LCHF diet are the same thing. While there are many similarities between these two diets, there are also some important differences and you will not get the same results from the Atkins diet as you will from the LCHF diet. To start with, when you are on the Atkins you will only need to limit the amount of carbs that you are eating during the induction period. As you proceed with the Atkins diet, you will be allowed to add more carbs back into your diet plan.

Not only will you be able to add the carbs back into your diet when you are on the Atkins plan, something that is not allowed on an LCHF diet, but you will also not be asked to pick fats that are high in quality. While on the Atkins diet, you can choose any fat that you want, such as margarines, saturated fats, and even oils that are rich in omega 6 acids. The Atkins diet is also not as strict in terms of the additives and preservatives that you can add in with your food compared to an LCHF diet. These are just some of the reasons why the Atkins diet will not be as successful for you as an LCHF diet.

When you are on the LCHF diet, you will be asked to limit your carb intake as much as possible. This limitation is not just for a couple of weeks and then you can put the carbs back into your diet. The carb limitation is something that is going to have to continue for the rest of your life. Doing this will force your body to use up the fat that is in it for energy, a state that is known as ketosis. In addition, the fats that you are allowed to eat on this diet must be of a high quality so that your body is able to efficiently use it as an energy source.

As you can see, there are some key differences that can be found between these three popular diet plans. Even though they all work with carbs in some way, they are quite different. Make sure that the rules that you are following match up with the LCHF diet if you want to see the best results.

Chapter 5—Recipes for the First 14 Days

Sometimes one of the most difficult things to do while on a new diet plan is to figure out what things that you should eat that are tasty and still remain true to the diet plan. This chapter is providing you with a menu for the first 14 days on the LCHF diet to help you to get started. Each day starts out with a breakfast, then a lunch, dinner, and finishes off with a dessert. Soon you will see how delicious and easy it is to follow this amazing diet plan!

Week 1

Monday

Gingerbread Muesli

Ingredients:

100 g. sunflower seeds
100 g. walnuts
100 g. almond flakes
100 g. chopped hazelnuts
6 tsp. gingerbread spice
3 Tbsp. coconut butter

Directions:

To begin this recipe, turn on the oven so that it can heat up to 350 degrees. Next, you can chop up all of the nuts before mixing them together in a bowl.

Take the coconut butter and melt it in the microwave before mixing it in a bowl along with the spice. Pour this melted butter on top of the nuts and mix together well.

Spread this nut mixture all over a baking tray before placing into the oven and letting it roast for 10 minutes. After this time, take it out and mix the nuts around. Place back into the oven and back for an additional 10 minutes.

Give the mixture some time to cool down and then enjoy!

Nutritional Facts:

Calories 189
Fat 15g
Carbs 2g
Protein 11g

Fried Halloumi

Ingredients:

2 eggs
½ c. almond flour
1 c. halloumi cheese
Pepper
Salt
Olive oil

Directions:

To begin this recipe, cut up the halloumi into slices before setting aside.

Bring out a bowl and whisk together the eggs. When the eggs are mixed, add in the pepper, salt, and almond flour.

Place the cheese in with this mixture and coat completely.

Heat up some oil in a frying pan before placing the cheese inside. Let it cook until it begins to turn brown and melt. Enjoy!

Nutritional Facts:

Calories 359

Fat 43g
Carbs 10g
Protein 0g

Creamy Thai Salmon

Ingredients:

2 salmon fillets
Thai curry paste
200 ml. cream
Salt
Pepper
Butter
½ head of cauliflower

Directions:

Start this recipe off by heating up the oven to 375 degrees. While the oven is heating up, use the butter to grease a baking dish and place the salmon inside.

Bring out a bowl to mix together the curry paste and cream, adding pepper and salt to taste. Pour this mixture on top of the salmon before placing into the oven.

Let the salmon bake for about 15 minutes. While the salmon is baking, grate up the cauliflower and fry it with some coconut butter until it becomes soft.

When the salmon is done cooking, serve it with the cauliflower and some thai sauce before enjoying.

Nutritional Facts:

Calories 267
Fat 12g
Carbs 2g
Protein 25g

Panna Cotta and Strawberries

Ingredients:

300 ml. cream
2 ½ gelatin leaves
2 Tbsp. sugar
1 lime zest
Juice from half a lime
200 ml. basil leaves
5 strawberries

Directions:

To begin this recipe, you can take the gelatin leaves and soak them in some water. While those are soaking. Bring out a saucepan and heat up the sugar and the cream. Make sure to stir to help the sugar dissolve.

Take the cream from the heat once it reaches a boil. Add in the basil and the lime zest before setting aside to cool down for 40 minutes.

After this time you can strain out the cream and then add in the lime juice. Slowly add the cream back in. Place the gelatin in and then stir to help dissolve.

Divide this mixture up among four molds before placing into the fridge overnight. Garnish with the basil and strawberries before serving.

Nutritional Facts:

Calories 210
Fat 14g
Carbs 5g
Protein 2g

Tuesday

Prawn Salad

Ingredients:

100 g. prawns
2 boiled eggs
1 chopped onion
Dill
4 Tbsp. mayo
Lime juice
Pepper
Salt

Directions:

Take the eggs and the onion and chop them into small pieces.

When this is done, bring out a bowl and mix them together along with the rest of the ingredients. Season with the pepper, salt, and dill how you like.

Enjoy right away.

Nutritional Facts:

Calories 210
Fat 23g
Carbs 4g
Protein 32g

Sushi

Ingredients:
Rice

75 g. butter
500 g. cauliflower
1 Tbsp. rice vinegar
Filling
1 avocado
160 g. cream cheese
200 g. salmon
Wasabi
Soy sauce
4 rice papers

Directions:

You can start this recipe by making the rice. To do this, take out a cheese grater and grate up the cauliflower. Place it into a frying pan with some butter and fry for about 10 minutes so it becomes creamy. Add in the vinegar and blend it well. Give the rice time to cool.

While the rice is cooling, cut up the avocado and salmon into thin slice. When you are ready, lay out the rice paper before spreading some cream cheese out on it.

Place the rice on top of the cream cheese before adding the avocado and salmon on top. Roll it up and cut into smaller pieces.

Serve the sushi with the soy sauce and wasabi

Nutritional Facts:

Calories 435
Fat 37g
Carbs 8g
Protein 20g

Meatballs

Ingredients:

400 g. pork
1 sliced garlic
1 sliced onion
1 egg
Pepper
Salt
Almond flour

Directions:

To begin this recipe you can chop up the garlic and the onion. Bring out a bowl and mix together the garlic and onion with the rest of the ingredients.

Using your hands, make 20 small meatballs with this mixture.

Roll the meatballs through the almond flour before placing them in a skillet with some butter. Cook until browned through before serving.

Nutritional Facts:

Calories 255
Fat 18g
Carbs 10g
Protein 19g

Chocolate Cake

Ingredients:

6 eggs
2 Tbsp. sugar
300 g. dark chocolate
½ c. cream
3 Tbsp. cold coffee

Coconut flakes

Directions:

Turn on the oven and let it heat up to 400 degrees. While that is heating up, you can use the butter to grease up the cake pan before setting aside.

Divide up the eggs and whisk together the whites. Place the chocolate into a bowl and let it melt in the microwave before mixing it with the egg yolks, coffee, and sugar.

Mix this chocolate mixture in with the egg whites slowly and continue mixing until it becomes smooth. Pour this batter into a pan and then into the oven.

Let the cake cook for about 10 minutes. When the cake is done, you can place into the fridge for an hour and then serve.

Nutritional Facts:

Calories 284
Fat 12g
Carbs 10g
Protein 3g

Wednesday

Vegetable Scramble

Ingredients:

2 eggs
4 cherry tomatoes
1 cucumber
Handful nuts
Olive oil

Directions:

Begin this recipe by taking the two eggs and scrambling them together in a skillet with some olive oil. Season with some pepper and salt when they are done.

While the eggs are cooking, chop up the tomatoes and cucumber before adding into the skillet along with the eggs.

Add the nuts last and serve right away.

Nutritional Facts

Calories 212
Fat 20g
Carbs 8g
Protein 23g

Sausage Gratin

Ingredients:

1 lb. sausage
1 c. broccoli
200 ml. cream
Pepper
Salt
Cayenne pepper
1 c. cheese

Directions:

Turn on the oven and let it heat up to 400 degrees. Take the broccoli and boil it for a few minutes, allowing it to become a little soft. Cut it up along with the sausage and place into a baking dish.

Mix the cream together with your cayenne pepper, salt, and pepper. Pour this mixture on top of the sausage and broccoli pieces.

Top with the cheese before placing the dish into the oven and letting it bake for about 30 minutes. Serve right away.

Nutritional Facts:

Calories 385
Fat 10g
Carbs 2g
Protein 23g

Veal Milanese

Ingredients:

4 pieces of veal
1 lemon
1 zucchini
Ground almond
Pepper
Salt
Butter
2 eggs

Directions:

Turn on the oven and let it heat up to 400 degrees. While that is heating up, you can cut the zucchini up and place into an oven dish. Season with the pepper and salt.

Place the dish into the oven and let them bake for 25 minutes. While the zucchini is baking, mix together the pepper, salt, and ground almond and set aside. Whisk together the eggs in another bowl.

Take the veal and put it into the egg bowl and then the ground almond mixture and then through the eggs again. Do this a couple times to get a crust.

Fry up the veal in a skillet, cooking it through. Serve the veal with your fried zucchini and some lemon.

Nutritional Facts:

Calories 459
Fat 34g
Carbs 5g
Protein 19g

Chocolate Mousse

Ingredients:

100 g. chocolate
2 eggs
½ c. cream
1 tsp. vanilla powder

Directions:

To begin this recipe, take the chocolate and break it into smaller pieces. Place into a bowl over some simmering water and allow to melt.

Bring out a bowl and whisk together the vanilla powder and egg. When the egg mixture is well combined, whisk it in with the chocolate.

In another bowl, whip the cream before folding it into the chocolate mixture until it just starts to combined.

Place this mixture into some bowls and let it set for a minimum of an hour so it can set.

Serve with some fruit and enjoy.

Nutritional Facts:

Calories 189
Fat 13g
Carbs 2g
Protein 2g

Thursday

Gorgonzola and Walnut Omelette

Ingredients:

½ c. gorgonzola cheese
2 eggs
¼ c. cream
Handful walnuts

Directions:

Put a little bit of oil onto a skillet and let it warm up. Add the eggs in next and let them fill up the pan. Allow the egg some time to cook.

Once the egg is almost done cooking, add in the cheese and some cream and let it cook for another minute more.

Add in the walnuts right before serving.

Nutritional Facts

Calories 334
Fat 19g
Carbs 5g
Protein 30g

Chicken Tacos

Ingredients:

1 taco mix packet
600 g. minced chicken
50 ml. water
Butter for frying
50 ml. cream
Toppings of your choice

Directions:

To start this recipe, fry up the chicken so that it is cooked all the way through.

Add the taco spice, cream, and water and mix it together, making sure to fry for an additional few minutes so it warms up.

While the chicken is cooking, grate the cheese and cut up the vegetables.

Serve the chicken with the cheese and top with your favorite toppings.

Nutritional Facts:

Calories 340
Fat 17g
Carbs 4.2 g
Protein 15g

Taco Burger

Ingredients:

1 egg
500 g. pork
50 ml cream
1 taco mix
Butter
50 ml. water

Directions:

Take the pork and mix it together with the taco spices, water, cream, and the egg, making sure to blend them up well.

Heat up some butter in the frying pan. Take your pork mixture and form it into four patties before adding into the frying pan. Fry for about 2 minutes on each side or until cooked through.

When the burgers are done, serve with a salad and some cheese before enjoying.

Nutritional Facts:

Calories 434
Fat 18g
Carbs 5g
Protein 15g

Coconut Pudding

Ingredients:

2 Tbsp. sweetener
3 eggs
300 ml. coconut flakes
100 ml. coconut cream
2 apples

Directions:

To start this recipe, you can turn on the oven and let it heat up to 350 degrees. While the oven is heating up you can prepare a water bath.

Bring out a bowl and mix together the coconut cream, sweetener, coconut flakes, eggs and then make a well inside the bowl. Pour this batter into a pan before placing into the prepared water bath before placing in the oven.

Bake for about 40 minutes so that the pudding begins to turn golden. While the pudding is cooking, you can core your apples before cutting them into small cubes.

Place the apples into a pot and turn the heat on low. Let the apples cook until they become a sauce, making sure to stir a few times.

Serve the apple sauce and the pudding together and enjoy.

Nutritional Facts:

Calories: 386
Fat 14g
Carbs 2g
Protein 3g

Friday

Porridge

Ingredients:

100 ml. coconut milk
2 eggs
Cinnamon
Vanilla powder
1 Tbsp. coconut flour
Cardamom

Directions:

Bring out a saucepan to begin this recipe and combine together all of the ingredients inside.

Allow the ingredients to come to boil before reducing to a simmer. Simmer for a few minutes until the desired consistency is met.

Serve this porridge with some berries or coconut.

Nutritional Facts:

Calories 154
Fat 12g
Carbs 10g
Protein 2g

Sausage Gratin

Ingredients:

1 lb. sausage
1 c. broccoli
200 ml. cream
Pepper
Salt
Cayenne pepper
1 c. cheese

Directions:

Turn on the oven and let it heat up to 400 degrees. Take the broccoli and boil it for a few minutes, allowing it to become a little soft. Cut it up along with the sausage and place into a baking dish.

Mix the cream together with your cayenne pepper, salt, and pepper. Pour this mixture on top of the sausage and broccoli pieces.

Top with the cheese before placing the dish into the oven and letting it bake for about 30 minutes. Serve right away.

Nutritional Facts:

Calories 385
Fat 10g
Carbs 2g
Protein 23g

Veal Milanese

Ingredients:

4 pieces of veal
1 lemon
1 zucchini
Ground almond
Pepper
Salt
Butter
2 eggs

Directions:

Turn on the oven and let it heat up to 400 degrees. While that is heating up, you can cut the zucchini up and place into an oven dish. Season with the pepper and salt.

Place the dish into the oven and let them bake for 25 minutes. While the zucchini is baking, mix together the pepper, salt, and ground almond and set aside. Whisk together the eggs in another bowl.

Take the veal and put it into the egg bowl and then the ground almond mixture and then through the eggs again. Do this a couple times to get a crust.

Fry up the veal in a skillet, cooking it through. Serve the veal with your fried zucchini and some lemon.

Nutritional Facts:

Calories 459
Fat 34g
Carbs 5g
Protein 19g

Ice Cream

Ingredients:

3 egg yolks
2 tsp. vanilla
300 ml. whipping cream
Flavoring of choice.

Directions:

Take out a bowl and mix together the vanilla, egg yolks, and the flavoring that you have chosen.

In another bowl you can whip up the cream before mixing in with the yolk mixture.

Pour this batter into your ice cream machine. Allow it to work until it reaches the consistency that you like. If you do not have an ice cream machine, you can pour into a pan and place nto the freezer for about 2 hours.

Serve right away.

Nutritional Facts:

Calories 211
Fat 10g
Carbs 2g
Protein 1g

Saturday

Cheese Muffins

Ingredients:

1 c. crème fraiche
2 eggs
25 g. butter
2 Tbsp. psyllium husk
¼ c. pumpkin seeds
¼ c. sunflower seeds
1 c. hard cheese
½ tsp. salt
1 tsp. caraway seed

Directions:

To begin this recipe, turn on the oven and let it heat up to 400 degrees. Next, separate out the yolk and the white from the egg and place them into different bowls.

Whisk the yolks together with the melted butter and the crème fraiche before adding in the salt, caraway, psyllium cheese, and seeds.

Next, whisk the egg whites until they are firm before folding in with the rest of the ingredients. Pour this batter into a muffin tin before placing into the oven.

Bake these muffins for about 15 minutes. Once they are done let them cool down before enjoying.

Nutritional Facts:

Calories 210
Fat 33g
Carbs 10g
Protein 5g

Cheese Pie

Ingredients:

Pie Shell
1 egg
50 g. butter
300 ml. ground almond
Filling
4 eggs
Pepper
Salt
200 ml. cream
150 g. mozzarella cheese
Olives
150 g. feta

Directions:

Turn on the oven and let it heat up to 400 degrees. Next, you can work on the pie shell. To do this, you can mix together the egg, butter, and ground almond. Place in a baking dish and let bake in the oven for about 8 minutes.

Chop up the olives, feta, and mozzarella cheese and mix together in a bowl. In another bowl, mix together the pepper, salt, cream, and eggs.

Put the olives and cheeses into the pie shell before topping the cream mixture on top. Place the pie back into the oven and let it bake for another 40 minutes.

Serve right away.

Nutritional Facts:

Calories 338
Fat 23g
Carbs 10g
Protein 5g

Tomato Chicken

Ingredients

1 lb. chicken legs
1 c. paste, sundried tomatoes
½ c. cream
Pepper
Salt
½ c. broccoli

Directions:

Heat up the oven to 400 degrees. Bring out an oven dish and place the chicken inside. In a separate bowl, mix the tomato paste together with the cream before pouring it on top of the chicken.

Season the chicken with the pepper and salt before placing into the oven and letting it cook for an hour or until the chicken is done.

When the chicken is almost done cooking, boil the broccoli. Serve with the chicken and enjoy.

Nutritional Facts:

Calories 410
Fat 20g
Carbs 3g
Protein 18g

Lemon Cake

Ingredients:

100 g. ground almonds
2 lemons
2 tsp. baking powder
100 g. ground coconut
2 Tbsp. sweetener
50 g. coconut oil
1 tsp. psyllium husk
Salt
3 eggs

Directions:

Turn on the oven and let it heat up to 350 degrees. While the oven is heating up, you can grease the cake pan up and set it aside. Grate your lemon peel next and squeeze out some of the juice.

In a bowl, you can mix together all of the dry ingredients. Taking out another bowl, mix together the liquid ingredients.

When both bowls are well mixed, pour the liquid mixture in with the dry ingredients before mixing well. Pour this batter inside a pan before placing into the oven.

Bake the cake for around 30 minutes. Allow some time to cool down before cutting into 8 pieces and enjoying.

Nutritional Facts:

Calories 218
Fat 22g
Carbs 11g
Protein 1g

Sunday
Morning Boost

Ingredients:

2 egg yolks
1 c. frozen raspberries
1 avocado
½ c. coconut milk
Vanilla powder

Directions:

To begin this recipe, bring out your blender and place all of the ingredients inside. Make sure to put the lid on top.

Mix the ingredients together for about a minute or until they become smooth and creamy.

Pour into your favorite glass and enjoy.

Nutritional Facts:

Calories 89
Fat 12g
Carbs 2g
Protein 10g
Tomato Chicken

Ingredients

1 lb. chicken legs
1 c. paste, sundried tomatoes
½ c. cream
Pepper
Salt
½ c. broccoli

Directions:

Heat up the oven to 400 degrees. Bring out an oven dish and place the chicken inside. In a separate bowl, mix the tomato paste together with the cream before pouring it on top of the chicken.

Season the chicken with the pepper and salt before placing into the oven and letting it cook for an hour or until the chicken is done.

When the chicken is almost done cooking, boil the broccoli. Serve with the chicken and enjoy.

Nutritional Facts:

Calories 410
Fat 20g
Carbs 3g
Protein 18g

Chicken Burger

Ingredients:

2 eggs
600 g. minced chicken
1 garlic clove
50 ml. cream

Pepper
Salt
Basil

Directions:

Bring out a bowl to start this recipe and mix together all of the ingredients.

Using your hands you can form the mixture into four patties before adding them into a skillet with some butter. Cook for two minutes on each side or until completely cooked.

Serve with some vegetables and enjoy.

Nutritional Facts:

Calories 287
Fat 22g
Carbs 6g
Protein 10g
Simple Cookies

Ingredients:

75g butter
2 ½ Tbsp. cocoa powder
150 g. ground almonds
1 egg white
1 tsp. vanilla
1 Tbsp. honey

Directions:

To begin this recipe, turn on the oven and let it heat up to 400 degrees. Next, you can bring out a bowl and place all of the ingredients inside. Mix until well combined.

Drop tablespoonfulls of the batter onto a prepared baking sheet and place into the oven. Let the cookies bake for about 10 minutes or until golden brown. Enjoy!

Nutritional Facts:

Calories 89
Fat 8g
Carbs 3g
Protein 2g

Week 2

Monday

Coconut and Raspberry Smoothie

Ingredients:

150 g. unsweetened raspberries
1 can coconut crème
Ice cubes
2 tsp. honey

Directions:

Bring out a mixing bowl and then through the sweetener, berries, and coconut crème inside. Make sure to mix it together thoroughly, mashing up the raspberries if you wish.

Pour this mixture out into a cup and add in the ice cubes. Enjoy right away.

Nutritional Facts:

Calories 112
Fat 10g
Carbs 1g

Protein 8g

Goulash Soup

Ingredients:

250 g. beef mince
1 yellow onion
1 carrot
1 red pepper
5 mushrooms
1 garlic clove
10 cherry tomatoes
200 ml. red wine
3 Tbsp. chicken stock
3 Tbsp. butter
1 tsp. paprika
1 tsp. caraway, crushed
1 tsp. Worcester sauce
Salt
300 ml. water
1 Tbsp. tomato puree
Pepper

Directions:

To start this recipe, dice up the onion, pepper, and carrot into smaller piece. Take the garlic and grate it as well.

Half the mushrooms and then slice them before cutting up the tomatoes.

Heat up your saucepan with a little bit of butter before frying up the beef. When the beef is cooked, add in the thyme, caraway, pepper, salt, garlic, and onion. Allow these to cook together for a few minutes.

Add in the pepper and the carrots and continue cooking to heat up before adding the mushrooms and tomatoes.

Next, add in the Worcester sauce, water, stock, and wine before bringing everything to a boil and letting it simmer for an hour.

Serve right away.

Nutritional Facts:

Calories 439
Fat 17g
Carbs 11g
Protein 18g

Tuna Cheese Casserole

Ingredients:

1 bell pepper, red
2 cans tuna
225 g. cottage cheese
75 g. hard cheese
Bunch of dill
Butter
Pepper
Salt
5 eggs

Directions:

To begin this recipe, turn on the oven and preheat it to 350 degrees. Use some of the butter to grease up a casserole dish and then set it aside.

Take the dill and the bell pepper and chop them up. Grate up the cheese, setting some of it to the side and drain out the tuna.

Mix all of the ingredients except the reserved cheese, into a bowl and season with some pepper and salt. Pour this mixture into the casserole dish and sprinkle with leftover cheese.

Place the dish into the oven and bake for about 40 minutes so that it can turn golden brown and set. Enjoy right away.

Nutritional Facts:

Calories 411
Fat 14g
Carbs 3g
Protein 10g

No Bake Cookies

Ingredients:

100 g. butter
1 c. almond meal
100 g. unsweetened coconut
2 Tbsp. coffee, strong
2 Tbsp. cocoa powder
Vanilla powder
50 ml. honey

Directions:

To begin this recipe, you can bring out a bowl and mix everything together using your hands. Take the dough and roll it into a log before placing into the refrigerator for about an hour.

After the hour is up, you can roll the log through some coconut before slicing it up and place into the fridge again. Enjoy when you are ready.

Nutritional Facts:

Calories 110
Fat 14g
Carbs 2g
Protein 0g

Tuesday

Berry Crisp

Ingredients:

1 c. blueberries
2 c. strawberries
¼ c. cornstarch
1 c. raspberries
4 tsp. sugar
1 c. rolled oats
5 Tbsp. butter
1/3 c. ground almond
½ c. stevia
½ tsp. salt
½ c. pecans
½ tsp. cinnamon

Directions:

To start this recipe you can turn on the oven to 350 degrees. While the oven is heating up, place the berries into a bowl. Toss the 4 teaspoons of sugar and cornstarch in with the berries before pouring into a baking dish.

Next, combine together the cinnamon, salt, pecans, stevia, almond, and oats. Dice the butter into the ixture so it becomes incorporated. Pour this on top of the berries and distribute.

Place into the oven and bake for about 35 minutes so that the top begins to brown. Enjoy right away.

Nutritional Facts:

Calories 198
Fat 17g
Carbs 10g
Protein 41g

Salmon Salad

Ingredients:

200 g. cherry tomatoes
3 red peppers
70g rucola
50 g. almond
120 g. chevre
600 g. smoked gallon
1 Tbsp. vinegar, white balsamic
4 Tbsp. olive oil
Pepper
Salt

Directions:

Preheat the oven to 250 degrees. While that is heating up, you can deseed the pepper and then cut into four pieces. Place the peppers onto an oven tray. Bake for 30 minutes so that the skin can start to bubble.

When the peppers are done, you can take them off the tray and into a plastic bag. Halve your tomatoes and toast the almonds before continuing.

Place the salad onto four plates and divide up the salmon on top of it. Top with the chevre cheese and the tomatoes along with the almonds and peppers.

Drizzle on some vinegar and olive oil and season with pepper and salt before enjoying.

Nutritional Facts:

Calories 264
Fat 10g
Carbs 1g
Protein 12g

Salami Pizza

Ingredients:

4 eggs
100 ml. coconut flour
100 ml. ground almond
Oregano
4 tsp. psyllium husk
Mozarella
Red pepper
Salami
Tomato paste
Salt
Pepper
Grated cheese

Directions:

To begin this recipe, turn on the oven to 400 degrees. Mix together all of the ingredients through the psyllium husk in a bowl.

Place the mix on a tray and spread it out to make a base. Place the tray into the oven and let it bake for about 7 minutes.

Take the base out of the oven and spread out the tomato paste all over it. Place the rest of the toppings over the pizza and then put it all bake back into the oven.

Bake the pizza for another 15 minutes before cutting into 8 pieces and serving.

Nutritional Facts:

Calories 318
Fat 22g
Carbs 4g
Protein 10g

Lime Truffles

Ingredients:

50 g. butter
300 g. dark chocolate
200 ml. cream
Salt
Peel of 1 lime

Directions:

To start this recipe, you can split the chocolate up into smaller pieces. Take the butter and cream and place into a pot and heat up. Add in the chocolate and then continuously stir until chocolate melts.

At this time, add in the lime peel and mix some more. Put this mixture into a dish before adding some salt on the top.

Place the dish into the refrigerator overnight. When you are ready to enjoy you can cut it up into small pieces and enjoy.

Nutritional Facts:

Calories 219
Fat 10g
Carbs 8g
Protein 2g

Wednesday

Sausage and Cheese Peppers

Ingredients:

20 jalapenos
10 oz. beef sausage, cooked
½ c. Parmesan
1 c. cream cheese

Directions:

Begin by turning on the oven and letting it heat up to 425 degrees.

Take the jalapeno peppers and cut them in half before deseeding them. Bring out a mixing bowl and combine the Parmesan cheese and the cream cheese together. Add in the sausage with this mixture.

Use this mixture to fill up the jalapeno peppers. Top with some more of the grated cheese. Place into a baking dish and then into the oven. Let it cook for 25 minutes so the peppers can become soft.

Take from the oven when done and enjoy!

Nutritional Facts:

Calories 226
Fat 21g

Carbs 3g
Protein 8g

Broccoli Soup

Ingredients:

Coconut oil
1 onion
2 c. water
500 g. broccoli
2 tsp. salt
2 Tbsp. whipping cream
Pepper
2 tsp. vinegar, white wine
2 ½ Parmesan cheese

Directions:

To begin this recipe, chop up the onion before frying it in a pan with some coconut oil. Once the onion has had time to brown, add in the water and bring to boil.

Add in the broccoli and let it cook so it can become soft. Add in the whipping cream at this time and continue to cook until the soup can get hot.

Season with the vinegar, pepper, and salt and cook until ready to eat. Pour the soup into some bowls and top with the Parmesan cheese before serving.

Nutritional Facts:

Calories 143
Fat 15g
Carbs 2g
Protein 1g

Turkish Lamb Hot Dish

Ingredients:

4 Tbsp. butter
300 g. leg of lamb
200 ml. aubergine
1 green pepper
1 red pepper
½ yellow onion
1 tsp. oregano
10 black olives
½ tsp. chili flakes
½ tsp. mint
Salt

Directions:

To begin this recipe, heat up two frying pans on the stove. In one pan, fry up the meat with some butter and the spices. In the other pan, fry up the vegetables.

When all of the ingredients are golden brown, you can mix together the two pans and let them cook together for a few minutes.

Before serving, garnish with some parsley and feta cheese before enjoying.

Nutritional Facts:

Calories 501
Fat 13g
Carbs 5g
Protein 33g

Ingredients:

200 g. ricotta cheese
4 eggs
125 g. butter
50 ml. coconut flour
250 ml. almond flour
1 Tbsp. stevia
2 tsp. baking powder
2 Tbsp. psyllium husk
2 Tbsp. ging+erbreadspiece

Directions:

Turn on the oven and let it heat up to 350 degrees. While the oven is heating up, you can whisk together the egg and the sugar substitute while also melting the butter.

Pour the ricotta cheese and butter in with the egg mixture. In another bowl, mix together all of the dry ingredients. Mix the two bowls together before pouring into a baking dish.

Bake the gingerbread for about 40 minutes. Cut into slices and serve right away.

Nutritional Facts:

Calories 198
Fat 12g
Carbs 5g
Protein 3g

Thursday

Belgian Waffles

Ingredients:

¼ c. ricotta cheese

¼ tsp. cinnamon
2 eggs
¼ tsp. nutmeg
3 packets Splenda
½ tsp. baking powder

Directions:

Turn on your waffle iron and let it heat up while you prepare the rest of the recipe.

Bring out a bowl and beat the eggs until they become fluffy and light. Add in the rest of the ingredients and continue beating until smooth.

Pour all of the batter into the waffle iron and let them cook until the waffles are done. Top with some butter and a little sugar free syrup and enjoy right away.

Nutritional Facts:

Calories 246
Fat 15g
Carbs 8g
Protein 20g

Oven Pancake

Ingredients:

150 g. cheese, grated
450 g. bacon
8 eggs
250 g. cottage cheese
150 ml. cream

Directions:

Turn on the oven so that it can heat up to 375 degrees. While the oven is heating up you can cut the bacon and spread it out on a tray.

Mix together the remaining ingredients before pouring on top of the bacon. Place the tray inside the oven and let it bake for 15 minutes.

Serve right away.

Nutritional facts:

Calories 432
Fat 34g
Carbs 5g
Protein 12g

Chicken Korma

Ingredients:

1 chicken breast
½ yellow onion
½ garlic clove
1 c. coconut cream
2 Tbsp. coconut oil
2 Tbsp. ground almond
1 tsp. turmeric
1 tsp. lemon juice
1 ml. ground cardamom
1 ml. cinnamon
White pepper
Salt

Directions:

Start this recipe by cutting up the chicken into small pieces, slicing the onion, and grating the garlic clove.

Heat up some oil on a pan before adding in the onion and the chicken. Cook so the chicken starts to heat through.

Use the cardamom, cinnamon, turmeric, garlic, white pepper, and salt to season the onions and chicken and continue cooking for another minute.

At this time, add in the lemon juice, coconut cream, and ground almond before letting everything thicken for a few minutes.

Serve right away with a salad and enjoy!

Nutritional Facts:

Calories 249
Fat 10g
Carbs 6g
Protein 13g

Gingerbread Truffles

Ingredients:+

100 ml. cream
200 g. dark chocolate
25 g. butter
1 tsp. honey
2 tsp. gingerbread spice.

Directions:

Take the chocolate and split it up into smaller pieces. Bring out pot and place the butter and cream inside. Heat these up before placing the chocolate inside and letting it melt.

Add the spice into the melted chocolate before placing the whole mixture inside the fridge for a few hours.

Once the chocolate has set, make it into small balls. Next, put the balls back into the fridge and let them cool down until you are ready to serve.

Nutritional Facts:

Calories 215
Fat 12g
Carbs 8g
Protein 5g

Friday

Breakfast Meatballs

Ingredients:

½ lb. shredded cheddar cheese
3 eggs
2 Tbsp. minced onion
32 oz. pork sausage
1 lb. ground beef

Directions:

To begin this recipe, turn the oven on and let it heat up to 350 degrees.

Bring out a bowl and combine together all of the ingredients, making sure to mix it thoroughly.

Roll the ingredients into balls before placing onto a baking sheet. You should be able to get between 50 to 60 meatballs from this recipe.

Bake in he oven for about 20 minutes or until completely cooked through. Enjoy!

Nutritional Facts:

Calories 313
Fat 25g
Carbs 1g
Protein 21g

Chicken Soup

Ingredients:

200 g. chicken breast
1 yellow onion
1 carrot
1 red pepper
3 Tbsp. butter
4 mushrooms
2 Tbsp. stock
1 c. water
½ c. coconut cream
Chili flakes
2 tsp. curry powder
Salt

Directions:

Start this recipe by slicing up the vegetables, mushrooms, and chicken into small pieces. Place the vegetables and chicken into a pan with some butter and let them cook. Spice with the chili flakes, salt, and curry powder.

When the chicken is cooked through, you can pour this mixture into a pan before adding the stock, coconut cream, water and mushrooms.

Bring this all to a boil before reducing the heat and letting it all simmer for about 10 minutes. Serve the soup warm.

Nutritional Facts:

Calories 162
Fat 12g
Carbs 1g
Protein 24g

Hamburgers

Ingredients:

2 eggs
500 g. meat
5 ml. salt
50 ml. olive oil
5 ml. pepper
Coconut oil
Sliced cheese
Onions
Tomatoes
Cucumber
Lettuce

Directions:

To begin this recipe, bring out a bowl and mix together all of the ingredients through the pepper. Place into the fridge for about 30 minutes.

Using your hands, form the mixture into 4 patties and place them on the grill to cook. You will want to cook for around 4 minutes on each side in order to cook through.

Serve the patties with the cheese, tomatoes, onions, cucumber, and lettuce.

Nutritional Facts:

Calories 286
Fat 22g
Carbs 8g
Protein 18g

Shortcake

Ingredients:

½ c. sugar
4 c. strawberries
Whipped cream
6 dessert shells

Directions:

To begin this recipe, take the sugar and pour it on top of the strawberries. Allow this to set for around 20 minutes before continuing.

After this time, mash up the strawberries until they are crushed. Pour them over a dessert cup and top with some cool whip before enjoying.

Nutritional Facts:

Calories 195
Fat 20g
Carbs 6g
Protein 3g

Saturday

Bacon and Egg Muffins

Ingredients:

5 tsp. hot sauce
½ c. Colby jack cheese
6 bacon slices
1 chopped tomato
¼ tsp. garlic powder
12 eggs
1 tsp. salt
1 tsp. pepper
4 Tbsp. green onion
½ c. onion

Directions:

Begin this recipe by turning the oven on to 350 degrees. Continue by bringing out a skillet and cooking the bacon until done. Make sure to drain the grease off.

Take out a bowl and beat the eggs before adding the hot sauce, garlic powder, pepper, salt, tomato, green onion, and onion. Stir in the cheese and bacon next.

Spoon this mixture into some muffin cups before placing into the oven. Let this bake for about 20 minutes so that the tops can set.

Serve right away and enjoy!

Nutritional Facts:

Calories 110
Fat 8g
Carbs 2g
Protein 9g

Battered Fillets

Ingredients:

100 g. cod
100 ml. sesame seeds
1 egg white
100 ml. nigella sativa seeds
White pepper
Salt
1 Tbsp. olive oil
2 Tbsp. butter

Directions:

Take the fish and slice it thinly before seasoning with salt and pepper on each side.

Bringing out a bowl, whip the egg white so it becomes frothy. Bring out another bowl and mix together the seeds in it.

Dip the fish into the egg whites first before dipping into the seed mixture, making sure the seeds cover all of the fish.

Place the covered fish onto a plate and then put into the refrigerator for about 30 minutes to help the seeds stick a little easier.

When the 30 minutes are done, fry up the oil and butter inside a pan and then add the fish. Cook for a few minutes on both sides until the fish is done cooking. Serve right away.

Nutritional Facts:

Calories 268
Fat 19g
Carbs 10g
Protein 34g

Shakshouka

Ingredients:

1 c tomatoes
2 bell peppers
2 onions
4 garlic cloves
1 tsp. tabasco
2 eggs
Olive oil
Salt

Directions:

To begin this recipe, peel the onions and garlic before chopping them up. Take the peppers and cut them into small strips. Cut the tomatoes into eights as well.

Next, take the olive oil and melt it in a skillet. Add in the peppers, garlic, and onions and sauté them for a few minutes before adding the seasoning and tomatoes. Cook for a few minutes so a thick sauce forms.

Once the sauce is thick you can crack the eggs into it and allow them to cook until done. Serve this dish right away and enjoy!

Nutritional Facts:

Calories 377
Fat 12g
Carbs 5g
Protein 2g

Peach Cobbler

Ingredients:

¼ c. bisquick, heat smart
½ c. milk
1 egg
1 tsp. splenda
8 oz. diced peaches

Directions:

To start, drain out the peaches before separating into 4 dessert cups. Turn the oven on so that it can heat up to 400 degrees.

In a bowl, combine together the Splenda, milk, bisquick, and egg and the pour some of this mixture over the peaches.

Bake the cobbler for about 15 minutes so that the top starts to turn brown. Serve right away with some whipped cream.

Nutritional Facts

Calories 81
Fat 12g
Carbs 13g
Protein 4g

Sunday

Apple Almond Muffins

Ingredients:

2 c. almond meal
1 c. applesauce
4 Tbsp. butter spread
4 eggs

1 Tbsp. cinnamon
1 tsp. allspice
1 tsp. cloves

Directions:

To begin, turn on the oven and let it heat up to 350 degrees. While that is warming up, place the butter into the microwave and let it melt.

Next, you ill want to mix together all of the ingredients in a mixing bowl before pouring out into some muffin tins that are prepared.

Place the muffin tray into the oven and let it cook for about 12 minutes or until done. Remove from the oven when done and give time to cool down before enjoying.

Nutritional Facts:

Calories 182
Fat 15g
Carbs 6g
Protein 7g

Ginger and Garlic Salmon

Ingredients:

2 salmon fillets
2 garlic cloves
5 centimeters ginger
2 red chilies
5 Tbsp. soy
2 Tbsp. sesame seed oil
Pepper
Salt

Directions:

To begin this recipe, you can turn on the oven and let it heat up to 400 degrees.

While the oven is heating up, mix together the pepper, salt, sesame seed oil, soy, chili, garlic, and ginger.

Place the salmon into a baking dish before spreading the marinade over it. Allow to marinate for a few minutes before placing into the oven.

Let the fish cook for about 15 minutes or until baked through. Serve with some vegetables or another favorite side dish.

Nutritional Facts:

Calories 366
Fat 13g
Carbs 4g
Protein 26g

Spareribs

Ingredients:

1 lb. spareribs
Salt
Pepper
Paprika
Cayenne pepper
Chili powder

Directions:

Begin this recipe by turning on the oven and letting it heat up to 350 degrees. Bring out a bowl and mix the spices together.

After making sure that the spareribs are completely dry, you can rub the spice mixtures on each side.

Place the ribs on a rack in the oven and then place into the oven. Let the ribs cook for about 45 minutes before turning the over and cooking for an additional 45 minutes.

Serve with your favorite sides and enjoy.

Nutritional Facts:

Calories 341
Fat 25g
Carbs 2g
Protein 45g

Apples and Granola

Ingredients:

2 Tbsp. granola
1 apple
¼ tsp. cinnamon
1 tsp. stevia

Directions:

Take the apple and dice it into large chunks. Place into a bowl and top with the cinnamon, stevia, and granola.

Place the bowl into the microwave and let it heat up for about a minute or until warm. Eat right away.

Nutritional Facts:

Calories 145
Fat 14g
Carbs 10g
Protein 3g

Conclusion

The LCHF Diet is a really easy diet plan for you to follow if you can just keep in mind to limit the amounts of carbs that you are eating and choose healthy fats to eat instead. By following this advice, you are forcing your body to not rely on carbs but fat as an energy source to get daily tasks done. This is a much better way to see the weight loss that you have always wanted.

That is how simple the LCHF diet really is. Limit the amount of carbs that you consume each day, increase the fat that you consume and you will never need to count calories or weigh your food again. You will be able to eat as much as you want until you get full and still see the weight melt away!

Use this guidebook to help get started on your weight loss goals today and be amazed at how easy it can be to have the pounds go away.

Printed in Great Britain
by Amazon.co.uk, Ltd.,
Marston Gate.